NATURE'S REMEDIES

EXPLORING THE MEDICINAL POTENTIAL OF FRUITS, VEGETABLES, AND MINERAL RESOURCES

HERBAL TREATMENTS FOR 59 DIFFERENT ILLNESSES

INTRODUCTION

The adage "Health is wealth" resonates across generations, underscoring the enduring importance of well-being. Through time, the emphasis on health has remained steadfast. Contemporary society witnesses diverse approaches to healthcare, influenced by traditional beliefs, religious convictions, educational insights, and more, all converging with the common goal of promoting a healthy life. Nevertheless, these methods exhibit various shortcomings, encompassing issues of efficiency, accessibility, financial burdens, and potential side effects.

Crucially, natural therapy emerges as a cornerstone in healthcare, leveraging the intrinsic benefits of fruits, vegetables, and mineral resources. It stands as the earliest, most efficient, and cost-effective form of healthcare, rooted in centuries of empirical experimentation and selection based on observed benefits. Plants, being rich sources of vitamins, minerals, and essential chemical components, form a reliable foundation for maintaining health. Nutritionists advocate for the daily consumption of fruits and vegetables due to their vital role in providing essential nutrients. Remarkably, every part of a plant possesses medicinal properties, offering a holistic approach where various ailments can find remedy through plant-based treatments.

TABLE OF CONTENT

28. Internal heat
29. Toothache (Children)
30. Toothache (Adult)
31. Vein
32. Whitlow
33. Heart Attack
34. Sleeplessness
35. Infertility (Man)
36. Infertility (Women)
37. Quick ejaculation
38. Cattarh
39. Hair Breakage
40. Bald Head
41. Running Stomach
42. Weak Erection
43. Eyes Sight
44. Natural family planning
45. Children convulsion
46. Burns
47. Baby in wrong position in the womb
48. Scabie/rashes
49. Waist pain/Chest pain
50. Fungi infections
51. Virginal discharge
52. Boil
53. Cataract
54. Burning Sensation
55. Throat problem
56. Hernia
57. Lost of voice
58. Man power
59. Prostate disorder

60. Hypertension/Stroke

1.   TYPHOID FEVER: Get unriped pawpaw, unriped pine-apple, grape, ginger, lime orange, sugar cane and lipton tea. Cut everything into pieces, boil with fermented corn water for one hour. take one glass cup 3 times daily for one week.

2.   STOMACH ULCER: Get 7-8 unriped plantain, peel them, cut them to pieces and pound to paste. Put everything inside a plastic container (1 gallon), fill it with water. Allow to ferment for three days. Take on cup 2 times per day.

3.   ASTHMA COUGH: Get mango seed from as much as you can get, cut into pieces and keep under the sun to dry. Grind to powder. Put one spoon of the powder into a glass cup of water, stir and drink. Once in a day for 3-4 weeks.

4.   CHOLERA: Take two teaspoons of salt and one teaspoon of sugar. Add on short of dry gin. Drink all as single dose.

5.   RHEMATISM/ARTHRISTIS: Get as many seeds of Avocado pear, cut into pieces and dry under the sun. Grind to pow-der. Mix with plenty of honey to form paste. Take one spoon 3 times daily until problem is over.

6.   KELOID: At the initial stage: Wah thoroughly and apply a mixture of lime orange juice and salt, two times a day for one week.

At advanced stage: Cut bumps open after washing and apply a mixture of sea butter and python's fat daily until bumps disappear.

7.   WORMS: Get 3 pieces of wonderful cola, cut into pieces, put in a bottle of lime juice. Take one spoon two times per day for 3-4 days.

8.   PNEUMONIA: Get a handful of Garlic, grind to extract the juice. Drink a spoon and use the juice to rob the chest and back.

9.   HIGH BLOOD PRESSURE: Get the seeds of avocado pear cut into pieces, dry under the sun and grind into powder. Take one spoon into your palp and drink once per day for 3 weeks.

10.   SEVERE COUGH: Get about 10 pieces of bitter cola, grind to powder, add half cup of pure honey. Take 2 spoons 3 times a day for 4 days.

11.   WHOOPING COUGH: Get 6 Pieces of native Apple, 3 bulbs of garlic, 10 pieces of lime orange. Boil with water. Tke half cup two times a day untile problem is over.

12.   TUBERCULOSIS: Get 20-25 pieces of bitter cola, ginger of equal quantity and 3 bulbs of garlic. Grind and add a bottle of pure honey. Take 1 spoons 3 times a day, for 1-2 months.

13. DIABETES: Get bitter leaf and scent leaves, squeeze into water add little lime orange juice, grinded garlic and small potash. Take one short twice per day.

14. EAR DISCHARGE: Get two spoons of lime juice, 1 spoon of honey and small salt mix together. Apply to the ear with wool.

15. APPENDICITIS: Get fresh aloe vera gel, add grounded garlic. Take one spoon of the mixture into a glass cup of warm water and drink once in a day intil problem is over.

16. GONORRHEA: Get 3-4 pieces of wonderful cola, Ginger and garlic, cut into pieces. Put all in a bottle with lime orange juice. Take 2 spoon everyday untile it is gone.

17. STAPHLOCOCCIS AURES: Get 2 pieces of aloe-vera cut into pieces, put everything (in one gallon) container, add one bottle of pure honey, fill the container with water take half cup 2 time daily.

18. WOMAN UNDER HARD LABOUR: Get some leaves of cochorus olitorus (Ewedu vegitable) squeeze into watery mixture take one glass cup. The baby will be delivered.

19. MEASLES: Get the soil from termite hill. Boil for one hour with water. Use the water to bathe the baby.

20. WOUNDS: Clean the wound, apply a mixture of your urine and ashes, then apply bandage.

21. PILE, INTERNAL: Get pawpaw leaves, scent leaves and bitter leaves, squeeze into water and drink half cup 2 times a day.

22. PILE (EXTERNAL) I.E. HEAMOROID: Fry about 10 lizard eggs with palm oil and apply to the anus with cotton wool overnight until problem is over.

23. MENSTURATION PROBLEM: Get 3-5 wonderful cola, ginger and garlic, cut into pieces, pour into a bottle of lime orange joice. Take 2 spoons 2 time in a day.

24. LOSS WEIGHT: Get some corn silk, boil with water and Lime orange juice. Drink 1 cup 2 time a day. Or eat plenty of cabbage everyday with a cup of grape orange juice

25. LOSS OF MEMORY: Eat plenty of wall nut everyday with a spoon of origina honey.

26. BLOOD BUILDING: Get some quantity of pumpking leaves and garden egg leaves, squeeze out the juice add milk and drink. Or boil the stem of Guinea Corn with water and drink.

27.   ENZEMA/RING WORM: Mix some native soap with grounded potash, add lime orange. Apply the mixture to the affected area after bathe.

28.   TEETHING PROBLEMS IN CHILDREN: Get a mixture of lime orange juice and honey (equal quantity). Take 1 teaspoon 3 times daily

29.   TOOTHACHE: Dissolve common salt in small quantity of petrol. apply to the teeth with cotton wool about 5 times daily.

30.   VEIN: Take 2 spoons of pure honey 2 times daily

31.   WHITLOW: Use your urine to wash the finger, apply palm kernel oil then cut lime orange into rings, insert to the finger overnight. Do this for 3-4 days.

32.   HEART ATTACK: Get 2 bulbs of Onions, 12 bulbs of garlic and 3-4 bottles of honey. Grind and mix together. Take 2 spoons 3 times daily

33.   SLEEPLESSNESS: Add 3 spoons of honey into a glass cup of milk. Take all at bed time.

34. MALE INFERTILITY (LOW SPERM COUNT):

Get large quantity of guava leaves, add water and filter. Drink one glass cup 3 times per day for 1 week. eat plenty of carrot and cucumber daily for 2-3 week.

35. INFERTITLITY IN WOMEN: Get sage weed. Boil the leaf and flower. Drink 1 cup two time daily.

36. QUICK EJACULATION: Get 3-4 fresh okro, slice them; Get dry okro seed about half cup. put all in an empty bottle. Add one bottle of Soda/tonic water. Allow for 2 days to ferment. Take one short 2 times daily.

37. CATTARH: Get wonderful cola, cut into pieces add lime orange juice. Take one spoon 3 times in a day.

38. HAIR BREAKAGE: Get 1 bottle of olive oil and one bottle of Honey. Mix together and warm on fire for few minutes. Use the mixture to wash your hair.

39. BALD HEAD: Grind bird pepper, pawpaw seed and mix with lime orange juice. Use the mixture to rub the head. Hair will grow.

40. RUNNING STOMACH: Get fresh palp, add small

water mix and drink it raw.

41. WEAK ERECTIOM: Get plenty of white onions. Grind and extract the juice, mix with equal quantity of honey. Take 2 spoons 3 times daily.

42. EYES SIGHT: Get Get some fresh tomato leaves, squeeze out the juice and apply to the eyes one drop per day or mix honey with water, equal quantity apply as eye drop.

43. NATURAL FAMILY PLANNING: Get some roots of cashew tree. Boil and add honey, take 1 cup per day after monthly period for one week before making love.

44. CHILDREN CONVULSION: Get one Onion, small Garlic and ginger. Grind all and mix with palm kernel oil. Give the child to drink and use the mixture as cream for the child.

45. FIRE/WATER BURNS: Rub the affected areas with pure honey.

46. BABY IN WRONG POSITION IN THE WOMB: Get plenty of Cochoru Oktorus (Ewedu Vegetable). Cook the leaves as usual and drink one tea cup 2 times per day for one week.

47. SCABIES/RASHES: Get some potash, and native soap,

mix with lime orange juice. Use the mixture to rub affected parts daily.

48. WAIST PAIN/CHEST PAIN: Get some seeds of avocado pear (english pear). Cut into pieces and sun dry. Grind to powder. Add one spoon to palp and drink once a day for 2-3 weeks.

49. FUNGI INFECTIONS: Get some quantity of scent leaves, squeeze out the juice and use to rub the affected parts.

50. VIRGINAL DISCHARGE: Get 3-5 pieces of wonderful cola, some ginger amd garlic. Grind all and add lime orange juice. Take 2 spoons 2 times daily.

51. BOIL: Get 2-3 white beans & small potash. Grind together and add red palm oil. Apply to the boil.

52. CATARACTS: Add equal quantity of water, coconut water and pure honey, mix together. Use the mixture as eye drop

53. BURNING SENSATION: Get fresh cow milk add pure honey and drink.

54.   THROAT PAIN: Eat small quantity of ginger continu-
ously.

55.   HERNIA: Get some leaves of casia alata, boil with water
and drink one glass cup daily.

56.   LOSS OF VOICE: Get some Okro, cut into pieces and
pound, add small water and honey; and drink it.

57.   MAN POWER: Grind plenty of white onion; Extract the
juice mix with equal quantity of honey. Take about 2 spoons 2 times
daily.

58.   PROSTRATE DISORDER: Get plenty seeds of date
palm, Grind to powder, Mix with honey. Take 1 spoon 2 times daily

59.   STROKE/HYPERTENSION: Get mistletoe leaves.
Dry them under the sun and grind to powder. Take one spoon into a
cup of hot water and drink 2 times daily.